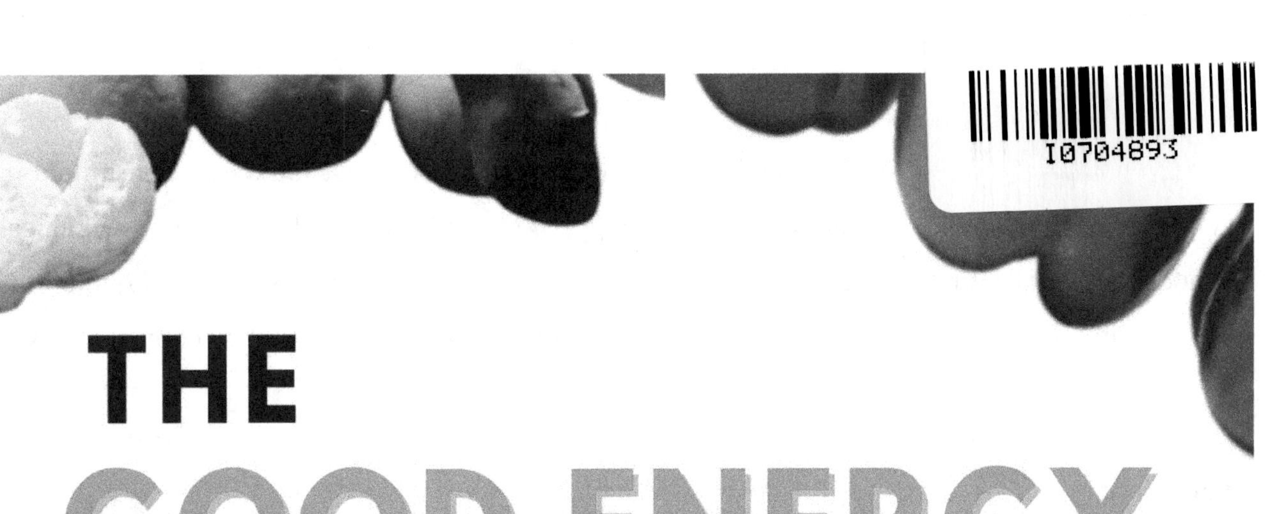

THE
GOOD ENERGY
Recipe Book

Transform Your Health, Boost Your Metabolism, Lose Weight, and Thrive with Over 140 Recipes, Perfect for Busy Professionals

BEATRICE R. KRAMER

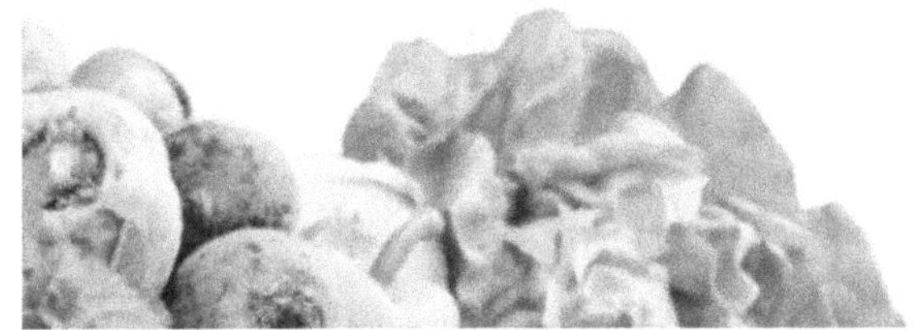

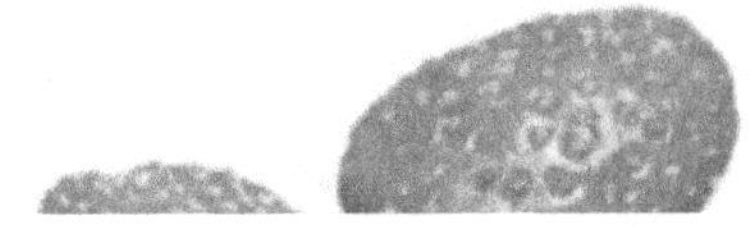

TABLE OF CONTENTS

In 2022, a growing number of health studies and discussions pointed to a powerful realization—our modern lifestyle was leaving us drained, tired, and unhealthy. In Portland, Oregon, health expert and doctor *Casey Means* published her groundbreaking research on how metabolism impacts chronic disease and overall health. Her work made it clear that the way our bodies process energy holds the key to unlocking better health and vitality.

With this in mind, this Good Energy Recipe Book is designed to build on those principles, helping you transform how your body functions on a cellular level. By focusing on whole foods, movement, and creating balanced meals, you can boost your metabolism and start feeling energized.

Drawing from the foundational work of *Dr. Casey Means* and her exploration of metabolic health, this recipe book will guide you in making practical, sustainable changes. The goal is to help you fuel your body the right way—through simple, nutrient-rich recipes that align with your body's natural processes.

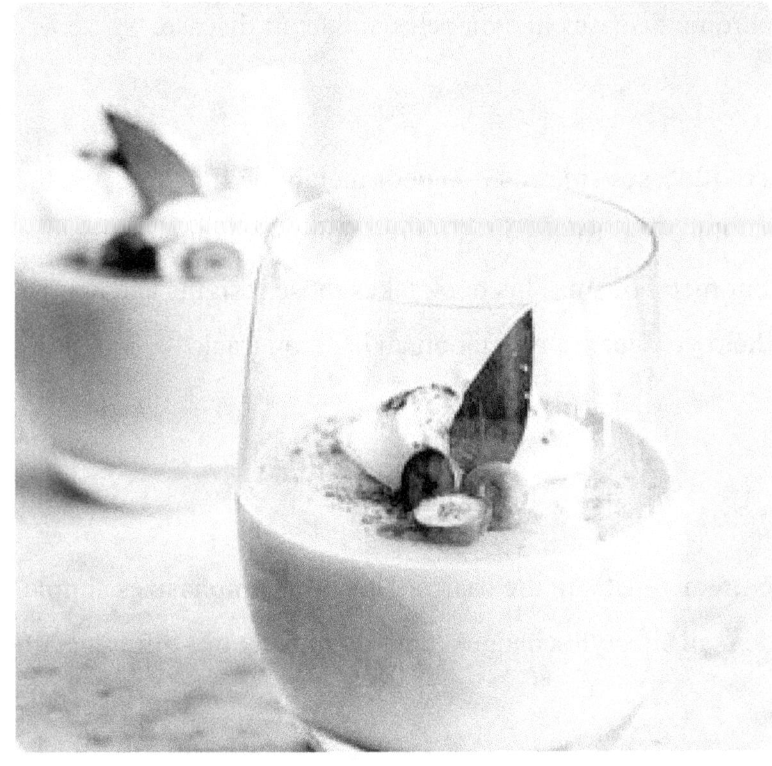

Chapter 1

Introduction to Good Energy Eating

Food is more than just fuel—it's the foundation for how our bodies create and maintain energy. Good Energy Eating focuses on meals that support optimal metabolic health, helping you feel vibrant and alive. The way we eat today often drains us, leaving us sluggish and prone to chronic illnesses. By choosing whole, nutrient-dense foods, we can transform our metabolism and improve overall well-being.

This book is designed to give you the tools to do just that. Through simple recipes and actionable tips, you'll learn how to eat in a way that boosts energy, supports metabolic function, and helps you thrive.

Understanding Metabolic Health And Why It Matters

Our metabolism is the engine that powers every cell in the body. When it runs smoothly, we have the energy to tackle each day with focus and strength. But when metabolic health is compromised, it can lead to weight gain, fatigue, and chronic diseases like diabetes and heart disease.

According to **Casey Means,** many modern illnesses are rooted in poor metabolic function, and the good news is that much of this is preventable. The food you eat, how you move, and even when you sleep all play a role in supporting your metabolism. This book takes those insights and applies them to real, everyday recipes that will help you get your metabolism back on track.

Food, Movement, and Lifestyle

The key to Good Energy isn't found in extremes—it's in the basics. This book emphasizes simple, balanced meals, regular movement, and small lifestyle changes that can make a big difference in how you feel.

a. Food: Choose whole, unprocessed foods that are rich in fiber, healthy fats, and proteins. Avoid refined sugars and processed snacks that spike blood sugar and lead to energy crashes.

b. Movement: Incorporate daily movement, whether it's a brisk walk, light stretching, or more intense exercise. Movement helps your cells use energy more efficiently.

c. Lifestyle: Good sleep, stress management, and spending time in natural light are crucial for maintaining energy levels. These simple habits can keep your metabolism functioning at its best.

By following these basics, you'll notice improvements in your energy, mood, and overall health. Each recipe in this book is designed with these principles in mind—balanced, easy to prepare, and focused on boosting your metabolic health.

Easy Steps to Get Started

If you're new to the world of Good Energy, don't worry small steps can lead to big changes. Here are a few easy ways to start improving your metabolic health:

a. Start with One Meal a Day: Focus on making one meal a day packed with whole foods. This could be a nutrient-dense breakfast or a balanced dinner. Each recipe in this book is designed to fit into your busy schedule.

b. Move for 10 Minutes a Day: You don't need to overhaul your exercise routine overnight. Start by moving for just 10 minutes a day   stretching, walking, or even dancing.

c. Hydrate: Drink water consistently throughout the day to help your metabolism run smoothly. You'll find drink recipes in this book to make hydration more enjoyable.

d. Sleep Well: Rest is crucial for energy. Create a bedtime routine to improve the quality of your sleep, whether that's winding down with a book or reducing screen time before bed.

e. Be Patient: Building Good Energy is a journey, and consistency is key. Focus on progress, not perfection.

This Good Energy Recipe Book is your guide to making sustainable, energy-boosting changes that fit into your lifestyle. Start with these small steps, and you'll be amazed at how quickly you begin to feel the difference.

Loved this book? There's more to explore!

If you enjoyed this book, I've got more in store for you! From healthy recipes to lifestyle tips, there's plenty to explore.

Simply scan the QR code below to discover more books from Beatrice R. Kramer.

Your next favorite read is just a scan away!

Chapter 2

The Core Principles of Good Energy

Understanding how your body uses energy is at the heart of improving health. Metabolic health, as Casey Means explains, is the foundation of good energy, vitality, and overall well-being. The core principles of Good Energy are centered on how you nourish your body with the right foods, how you balance those foods, and how you approach eating itself. In this section, you'll learn practical strategies to integrate these principles into your daily routine.

Whole Foods First

One of the most significant shifts you can make to improve your energy is to prioritize whole, unprocessed foods. Processed foods are loaded with refined sugars, unhealthy fats, and preservatives that disrupt your metabolism and lead to energy crashes.

Whole foods, on the other hand, are packed with the nutrients your body needs to function properly. As Casey Means emphasizes, our cells were designed to process foods in their natural state. When you fuel your body with whole foods like vegetables, fruits, lean proteins, and healthy fats, you give your cells the raw materials they need to produce energy efficiently.

How to Avoid Processed Foods

- Read Labels: Avoid foods with long ingredient lists or those containing ingredients you can't pronounce.
- Shop the Perimeter: Stick to the outer aisles of the grocery store, where fresh produce, meats, and whole grains are found.
- Cook at Home: Preparing your own meals gives you complete control over the ingredients.

Balanced Meals: Protein, Healthy Fats, and Fiber

A key principle of Good Energy is creating balanced meals that contain a combination of protein, healthy fats, and fiber. This trio works together to keep your blood sugar stable, prevent energy crashes, and fuel your body throughout the day.

- Protein: Supports muscle repair, immune function, and keeps you full. Include sources like lean meats, eggs, legumes, and nuts.
- Healthy Fats: Essential for brain function and long-lasting energy. Opt for fats from avocados, olive oil, and fatty fish like salmon.
- Fiber: Slows digestion and stabilizes blood sugar. Fill your plate with fiber-rich vegetables, fruits, and whole grains.

When you balance your meals, your body absorbs nutrients more effectively, providing steady energy and avoiding spikes in blood sugar. Each recipe in this book is crafted with this balance in mind, making it easy to enjoy satisfying, energy-boosting meals.

Listening to Your Body's Signals

In our fast-paced world, we often eat out of habit or convenience, ignoring the natural hunger and fullness signals our bodies give us. Mindful eating is about tuning into those signals and eating with intention.

Casey Means highlights the importance of reconnecting with your body's cues. Instead of eating on autopilot, mindful eating encourages you to slow down, savor each bite, and recognize when you're satisfied. This practice not only helps you enjoy your meals more but also prevents overeating and supports your metabolism.

Tips for Mindful Eating:

- Slow Down: Take your time when eating, chew thoroughly, and savor each bite.
- Listen to Hunger Cues: Eat when you're hungry, not out of boredom or routine.
- Stop When Full: Pay attention to when your body signals that it's satisfied and avoid overeating.

By incorporating mindful eating into your routine, you'll begin to develop a healthier relationship with food, and your body will naturally respond by feeling more energized and balanced.

Chapter 3

Meal Timing and Light Exposure

Our bodies function in sync with natural rhythms—circadian rhythms, to be precise—that regulate everything from digestion to sleep patterns. As Casey Means explains, when you eat and how you expose yourself to light significantly impacts your energy levels and metabolic health. This section will help you understand how to time your meals and manage light exposure to optimize energy production and overall well-being.

When to Eat: Aligning with Your Body's Clock

Your body's internal clock, known as the circadian rhythm, governs your energy cycles throughout the day. Eating in alignment with this natural rhythm can improve your metabolism and support good energy. Casey Means emphasizes the importance of not only what you eat but when you eat.

Eating during daylight hours, when your body is primed for digestion, allows your metabolism to function more efficiently. Conversely, late-night eating can disrupt your circadian rhythm, leading to poor energy levels and even weight gain.

Key Tips for Meal Timing:

- Start with Breakfast: Eating a well-balanced breakfast within a few hours of waking up helps jumpstart your metabolism for the day.
- Time Your Last Meal: Aim to finish your last meal at least 2-3 hours before bedtime. This allows your body to enter a restful state without having to focus on digestion.
- Eat During Daylight Hours: Keep your meals within a 12-hour window, ideally during daylight, to support your body's natural rhythms.

Aligning your meals with your body's clock means eating in tune with when your metabolism is most active, resulting in more consistent energy throughout the day.

How Light Affects Energy

Light exposure plays a crucial role in regulating your circadian rhythm and overall metabolic health. According to Casey Means, exposure to natural light, especially in the morning, helps synchronize your body's internal clock, while too much artificial light—particularly in the evening—can disrupt your energy cycles.

By controlling your exposure to light, you can influence how alert and energized you feel. Natural sunlight stimulates the production of serotonin, a hormone that keeps you awake and focused. Conversely, exposure to artificial light late at night can suppress melatonin production, making it harder to fall asleep and affecting your energy levels the next day.

Practical Light Exposure Tips:

Get Morning Sunlight: Spend at least 10-15 minutes outside in natural light after waking up. This helps reset your circadian rhythm and boosts your energy for the day.

Limit Blue Light at Night: Reduce exposure to screens (phones, laptops, etc.) in the hour or two before bed. Use warm lighting or blue light filters to minimize disruption to your sleep cycle.

Create a Sleep-Friendly Environment: Keep your bedroom dark and cool to enhance melatonin production, which promotes better sleep and helps you wake up feeling refreshed.

Incorporating these simple light management practices can significantly improve your sleep quality and daytime energy levels.

Chapter 4

Movement and Sleep for Better Energy

Movement and sleep are two essential pillars of metabolic health and overall energy. As Casey Means explains, the body's ability to produce energy efficiently is greatly influenced by how much you move during the day and how well you rest at night. This section outlines simple strategies to incorporate regular movement into your routine and create a sleep-friendly environment that supports long-term energy and vitality.

Simple Exercises to Boost Metabolism

Movement is a powerful tool to boost your metabolism and maintain steady energy levels. Regular physical activity stimulates your cells to produce more energy, improving both physical and mental well-being. Casey Means highlights the importance of incorporating even small amounts of movement into your day, as it helps your body burn fuel more efficiently and reduces metabolic dysfunction.

You don't need to engage in intense workouts to see benefits. Simple, consistent movement, such as walking, stretching, or light resistance exercises, can make a big impact on how your body produces and uses energy

Key Movement Tips:

- Take Short Walks: Walking for 10-15 minutes after meals helps regulate blood sugar and supports metabolism. Incorporating short walks throughout the day can make a big difference.
- Stretch or Do Light Yoga: Gentle stretching or yoga helps improve circulation and supports energy flow throughout the body.

- Use Body Weight Exercises: Exercises like squats, lunges, and push-ups are easy to do at home and help build muscle, which boosts metabolic health.

Creating a Sleep-Friendly Routine

Sleep is when your body does the important work of recovering, repairing, and recharging. According to Casey Means, poor sleep disrupts metabolic processes, leading to fatigue, weight gain, and even chronic illness. Quality sleep is crucial for maintaining balanced energy levels and optimal health.

Creating a sleep-friendly routine is essential to ensure you get the rest your body needs. Establishing consistent sleep patterns, minimizing exposure to artificial light before bed, and creating a calming environment can all contribute to better sleep quality.

Key Tips for Better Sleep:

- Stick to a Regular Schedule: Going to bed and waking up at the same time every day helps regulate your body's internal clock, making it easier to fall asleep and wake up energized.
- Create a Relaxing Bedtime Routine: Engage in calming activities, such as reading, meditating, or taking a warm bath, to signal to your body that it's time to wind down.
- Limit Caffeine and Electronics: Avoid caffeine in the late afternoon and reduce screen time before bed to prevent disruptions to your sleep cycle.

By focusing on rest and recovery, you'll wake up feeling refreshed, with more energy to tackle the day. Proper sleep, along with consistent movement, creates a solid foundation for metabolic health and overall vitality.

Chapter 5

Good Energy Recipes

Breakfast Recipes

Green Energy Smoothie

Time: 5 minutes

Serves: 2

Packed with leafy greens and healthy fats, this smoothie supports metabolism and offers long-lasting energy.

Ingredients:

- 2 cups spinach
- 1/2 avocado
- 1 banana
- 1 tablespoon chia seeds
- 1 cup unsweetened almond milk
- 1/2 teaspoon spirulina (optional)

Instructions:

1. Add all ingredients to a blender.
2. Blend until smooth and creamy.
3. Pour into glasses and enjoy.

Berry Protein Boost Smoothie

Time: 5 minutes

Serves: 2

A protein-rich smoothie featuring antioxidant-packed berries to kickstart your day.

Ingredients:

- 1/2 cup mixed berries (blueberries, raspberries, strawberries)
- 1 scoop plant-based protein powder
- 1 tablespoon flaxseeds
- 1/2 cup Greek yogurt (optional for extra protein)
- 1 cup water or almond milk

Instructions:

1. Place all ingredients in a blender.
2. Blend until smooth.
3. Serve chilled.

Tropical Energy Smoothie

Time: 5 minutes

Serves: 2

A tropical blend of fruits with a touch of coconut for a refreshing, energy-boosting start.

Ingredients:

- 1/2 cup pineapple chunks
- 1/2 cup mango
- 1/2 banana
- 1 tablespoon coconut oil
- 1 cup coconut water

Instructions:

1. Blend all ingredients until smooth.
2. Pour into glasses and enjoy fresh.

Chocolate Almond Energy Smoothie

Time: 5 minutes

Serves: 2

A rich and satisfying smoothie with almond butter and cacao to boost energy and mood.

Ingredients:

- 1 tablespoon almond butter
- 1 tablespoon raw cacao powder
- 1 banana
- 1 scoop plant-based protein powder
- 1 cup unsweetened almond milk

Instructions:

1. Add all ingredients to the blender.
2. Blend until creamy and smooth.
3. Serve immediately.

Matcha Power Smoothie

Time: 5 minutes

Serves: 2

This smoothie combines matcha's energizing properties with the creaminess of coconut milk for a metabolism-boosting drink.

Ingredients:

- 1 teaspoon matcha powder
- 1/2 avocado
- 1 tablespoon chia seeds
- 1/2 banana
- 1 cup coconut milk

Instructions:

1. Blend all ingredients until smooth.
2. Pour into glasses and enjoy.

Cinnamon Oat Energy Smoothie

Time: 5 minutes

Serves: 2

A fiber-packed smoothie with the warming flavor of cinnamon, great for a filling breakfast.

Ingredients:

- 1/4 cup rolled oats
- 1 banana
- 1/2 teaspoon cinnamon
- 1 tablespoon almond butter
- 1 cup oat milk

Instructions:

1. Combine all ingredients in a blender.
2. Blend until smooth.
3. Serve fresh and chilled.

Avocado Coconut Smoothie

Time: 5 minutes

Serves: 2

A creamy, nutrient-rich smoothie filled with healthy fats to fuel your metabolism.

Ingredients:

- 1/2 avocado
- 1/2 cup coconut milk
- 1 tablespoon chia seeds
- 1/2 banana
- 1 cup water or coconut water

Instructions:

1. Add all ingredients to the blender.

2. Blend until smooth.

3. Serve chilled.

Peach Mango Metabolism Booster

Time: 5 minutes

Serves: 2

This refreshing smoothie combines peaches and mangoes for a vitamin-packed, energizing drink.

Ingredients:

- 1/2 cup peach slices
- 1/2 cup mango
- 1 tablespoon ground flaxseeds
- 1 scoop protein powder
- 1 cup almond milk

Instructions:

1. Add all ingredients to a blender.
2. Blend until smooth.
3. Serve immediately.

Blueberry Chia Energy Smoothie

Time: 5 minutes

Serves: 2

Antioxidant-rich blueberries and fiber-packed chia seeds for a metabolism-friendly smoothie.

Ingredients:

- 1/2 cup blueberries
- 1 tablespoon chia seeds
- 1/2 banana
- 1 scoop protein powder

- 1 cup water or almond milk

Instructions:

1. Blend all ingredients until smooth.
2. Serve chilled and enjoy.

Green Detox Smoothie

Time: 5 minutes

Serves: 2

A detoxifying smoothie filled with greens and fresh herbs to start your day with clarity and energy.

Ingredients:

- 2 cups kale
- 1/4 cup parsley
- 1/4 cup cucumber
- 1 tablespoon flaxseeds
- 1 cup water or coconut water

Instructions:

1. Blend all ingredients until smooth.
2. Pour and serve immediately.

All smoothies can be stored in an airtight container for up to 24 hours in the refrigerator, but they are best enjoyed fresh to retain maximum nutrients and flavor.

Egg-Based Meals

Spinach and Feta Scramble

Time: 10 minutes

Serves: 2

A nutrient-packed scramble with spinach and feta for a high-protein, energy-boosting breakfast.

Ingredients:

- 4 eggs
- 1 cup fresh spinach
- 1/4 cup crumbled feta
- 1 tablespoon olive oil
- Salt and pepper to taste

Instructions:

1. Heat olive oil in a pan over medium heat.
2. Add spinach and cook until wilted.
3. In a bowl, whisk eggs with salt and pepper, then pour into the pan.
4. Stir until eggs are cooked through.
5. Top with crumbled feta and serve immediately.

Avocado Egg Toast

Time: 5 minutes

Serves: 1

Simple yet satisfying, this dish pairs protein-packed eggs with healthy fats from avocado.

Ingredients:

1 slice whole grain bread, toasted

1/2 avocado, mashed

2 poached eggs

Salt, pepper, and red pepper flakes to taste

Instructions:

1. Spread mashed avocado on the toasted bread.
2. Top with poached eggs.

3. Sprinkle with salt, pepper, and red pepper flakes for extra flavor. Serve immediately.

Veggie Omelet

Time: 10 minutes

Serves: 2

A protein-rich omelet packed with fiber from fresh vegetables for sustained energy.

Ingredients:

- 4 eggs
- 1/2 cup diced bell peppers
- 1/4 cup chopped onions
- 1/4 cup sliced mushrooms
- 1 tablespoon olive oil
- Salt and pepper to taste

Instructions:

1. Heat olive oil in a skillet over medium heat.
2. Add vegetables and sauté until tender.
3. Whisk eggs with salt and pepper, then pour into the skillet.
4. Cook until eggs are firm, fold, and serve.

Baked Egg Cups

Time: 15 minutes

Serves: 4

Perfect for meal prep, these baked egg cups provide a portable, protein-packed breakfast.

Ingredients:

- 8 eggs
- 1/2 cup diced bell peppers
- 1/2 cup chopped spinach

- 1/4 cup shredded cheese (optional)
- Salt and pepper to taste

Instructions:

1. Preheat oven to 350°F (175°C).
2. Grease a muffin tin and divide the vegetables evenly among the cups.
3. Whisk the eggs with salt and pepper, then pour over the veggies.
4. Top with cheese if using, and bake for 12-15 minutes.
5. Store in the fridge for up to 3 days.

Shakshuka

Time: 20 minutes

Serves: 2

A delicious, high-protein meal with poached eggs in a spiced tomato sauce.

Ingredients:

- 4 eggs
- 1 can (14 oz) crushed tomatoes
- 1/2 onion, diced
- 1 bell pepper, diced
- 1 clove garlic, minced
- 1 teaspoon cumin
- 1 tablespoon olive oil
- Salt and pepper to taste

Instructions:

1. Heat olive oil in a skillet over medium heat.
2. Sauté onion, bell pepper, and garlic until softened.
3. Add cumin and tomatoes, simmer for 10 minutes.
4. Make wells in the sauce and crack eggs into each.
5. Cover and cook until eggs are set, about 5 minutes. Serve hot.

Egg Muffins with Kale and Sweet Potatoes

Time: 25 minutes

Serves: 4

These savory muffins combine eggs, kale, and sweet potatoes for a nutrient-dense, high-protein breakfast.

Ingredients:

- 6 eggs
- 1 cup cooked sweet potatoes, diced
- 1 cup chopped kale
- 1 tablespoon olive oil
- Salt and pepper to taste

Instructions:

1. Preheat oven to 350°F (175°C).
2. Sauté kale in olive oil until wilted.
3. Whisk eggs with salt and pepper, and stir in sweet potatoes and kale.
4. Pour mixture into greased muffin tins and bake for 20 minutes.
5. Store in an airtight container for up to 3 days.

Egg and Veggie Stir-Fry

Time: 10 minutes

Serves: 2

A quick and easy stir-fry with scrambled eggs and vegetables, great for boosting metabolism.

Ingredients:

- 4 eggs
- 1/2 cup chopped broccoli
- 1/2 cup sliced mushrooms

- 1 tablespoon olive oil

- Salt, pepper, and soy sauce to taste

Instructions:

1. Heat olive oil in a skillet over medium heat.

2. Sauté broccoli and mushrooms until tender.

3. Whisk eggs and pour into the skillet.

4. Scramble eggs with the vegetables, season with salt, pepper, and a splash of soy sauce. Serve hot.

Egg and Salmon Breakfast Bowl

Time: 10 minutes

Serves: 1

A high-protein breakfast bowl featuring smoked salmon, eggs, and healthy fats for sustained energy.

Ingredients:

- 2 eggs, scrambled

- 2 oz smoked salmon

- 1/2 avocado, sliced

- 1/4 cup cooked quinoa

- Salt and pepper to taste

Instructions:

1. Scramble the eggs over medium heat.

2. Arrange the quinoa, smoked salmon, and avocado in a bowl.

3. Top with scrambled eggs, season, and serve.

Mexican Breakfast Tacos

Time: 10 minutes

Serves: 2

These breakfast tacos pack protein with scrambled eggs, black beans, and avocado for a hearty morning meal.

Ingredients:

- 4 eggs, scrambled
- 1/2 cup black beans
- 1/2 avocado, sliced
- 4 small corn tortillas
- Salsa and cilantro for garnish

Instructions:

1. Heat tortillas in a skillet.
2. Scramble eggs and heat black beans in a separate pan.
3. Divide eggs and beans among the tortillas, top with avocado slices, salsa, and cilantro. Serve immediately.

Egg White Veggie Frittata

Time: 20 minutes

Serves: 4

A light and protein-packed frittata with egg whites and mixed vegetables for a healthy start.

Ingredients:

- 8 egg whites
- 1/2 cup diced bell peppers
- 1/2 cup chopped spinach
- 1/4 cup chopped onions
- 1 tablespoon olive oil
- Salt and pepper to taste

Instructions:

1. Preheat oven to 350°F (175°C).

2. Sauté vegetables in olive oil until tender.

3. Whisk egg whites with salt and pepper, and pour over vegetables in the pan.

4. Cook on the stove for 2 minutes, then transfer to the oven and bake for 10-12 minutes until set. Serve hot.

Classic Almond Butter Oatmeal

Time: 10 minutes

Serves: 2

A creamy bowl of oats topped with almond butter for added protein and healthy fats.

Ingredients:

- 1 cup rolled oats
- 2 cups unsweetened almond milk
- 2 tablespoons almond butter
- 1 tablespoon chia seeds
- 1 teaspoon cinnamon

Instructions:

1. In a saucepan, bring almond milk to a simmer.

2. Stir in oats and chia seeds, and cook for 5-7 minutes until thickened.

3. Remove from heat and stir in cinnamon. Top with almond butter and serve warm.

Berry and Flax Oatmeal

Time: 10 minutes

Serves: 2

Rich in antioxidants and fiber, this oatmeal combines fresh berries and ground flax for a wholesome breakfast.

Ingredients:

- 1 cup rolled oats
- 2 cups water or almond milk
- 1/2 cup mixed berries (blueberries, raspberries)
- 1 tablespoon ground flaxseeds
- 1 tablespoon honey (optional)

Instructions:

1. Cook oats in water or almond milk over medium heat for 5-7 minutes.
2. Stir in flaxseeds and berries.
3. Drizzle with honey if desired, and serve.

Banana Walnut Oatmeal

Time: 10 minutes

Serves: 2

This hearty oatmeal is packed with potassium from bananas and omega-3s from walnuts.

Ingredients:

- 1 cup rolled oats
- 2 cups almond milk
- 1 banana, sliced
- 1/4 cup chopped walnuts
- 1 teaspoon cinnamon

Instructions:

1. Heat almond milk in a pot and stir in oats.
2. Cook for 5-7 minutes, then remove from heat.
3. Stir in banana slices, walnuts, and cinnamon. Serve warm.

Apple Cinnamon Oatmeal

Time: 10 minutes

Serves: 2

A warm, spiced oatmeal featuring apples and cinnamon for a comforting, fiber-rich meal.

Ingredients:

- 1 cup rolled oats
- 2 cups water or almond milk
- 1 apple, diced
- 1 teaspoon cinnamon
- 1 tablespoon chia seeds

Instructions:

1. Cook oats and water or almond milk in a saucepan.
2. Stir in apples, chia seeds, and cinnamon while cooking for an additional 2-3 minutes.
3. Serve with extra cinnamon on top.

Peanut Butter and Banana Oatmeal

Time: 10 minutes

Serves: 2

A protein-packed oatmeal with peanut butter and banana for sustained energy throughout the morning.

Ingredients:

- 1 cup rolled oats
- 2 cups almond milk
- 2 tablespoons peanut butter
- 1 banana, sliced
- 1 teaspoon vanilla extract

Instructions:

1. Heat almond milk in a saucepan and add oats.
2. Cook for 5-7 minutes until thickened, then stir in peanut butter and vanilla.
3. Top with banana slices and serve warm.

Coconut and Chia Oatmeal

Time: 10 minutes

Serves: 2

Creamy coconut milk and chia seeds make this oatmeal rich in healthy fats and fiber for a balanced start to the day.

Ingredients:

- 1 cup rolled oats
- 1 cup coconut milk
- 1 cup water
- 1 tablespoon chia seeds
- 1 tablespoon shredded coconut

Instructions:

1. Cook oats, coconut milk, and water in a saucepan for 5-7 minutes.
2. Stir in chia seeds and shredded coconut, then remove from heat.
3. Serve with a sprinkle of extra coconut on top.

Chocolate Hazelnut Oatmeal

Time: 10 minutes

Serves: 2

A decadent oatmeal made with raw cacao and hazelnuts for an energizing, antioxidant-rich breakfast.

Ingredients:

- 1 cup rolled oats
- 2 cups almond milk
- 1 tablespoon raw cacao powder
- 1/4 cup chopped hazelnuts
- 1 tablespoon honey (optional)

Instructions:

1. Heat almond milk and oats in a pot, cooking for 5-7 minutes.
2. Stir in cacao powder and hazelnuts, then remove from heat.
3. Sweeten with honey if desired, and serve.

Pumpkin Spice Oatmeal

Time: 10 minutes

Serves: 2

This fall-inspired oatmeal uses pumpkin puree and warm spices for a comforting, nutritious bowl.

Ingredients:

- 1 cup rolled oats
- 2 cups water or almond milk
- 1/4 cup pumpkin puree
- 1 teaspoon cinnamon
- 1/4 teaspoon nutmeg

Instructions:

1. Cook oats and liquid in a saucepan over medium heat for 5 minutes.
2. Stir in pumpkin puree, cinnamon, and nutmeg, cooking for an additional 2 minutes.
3. Serve warm with a sprinkle of cinnamon on top.

Blueberry Almond Oatmeal

Time: 10 minutes

Serves: 2

This energizing oatmeal combines blueberries and almonds for a fiber-rich, protein-packed breakfast.

Ingredients:

- 1 cup rolled oats
- 2 cups almond milk
- 1/2 cup fresh blueberries
- 1/4 cup sliced almonds
- 1 tablespoon ground flaxseeds

Instructions:

1. Heat almond milk and oats in a saucepan, cooking for 5-7 minutes.
2. Stir in blueberries, almonds, and flaxseeds.
3. Serve warm.

Maple Pecan Oatmeal

Time: 10 minutes

Serves: 2

Sweetened with pure maple syrup and topped with crunchy pecans, this oatmeal offers a perfect balance of carbs and healthy fats.

Ingredients:

- 1 cup rolled oats
- 2 cups water
- 1 tablespoon pure maple syrup
- 1/4 cup chopped pecans
- 1/2 teaspoon vanilla extract

Instructions:

1. Cook oats and water in a saucepan for 5-7 minutes.

2. Stir in maple syrup, vanilla extract, and pecans.

3. Serve warm with extra maple syrup if desired.

These oatmeal recipes follow Good Energy principles, providing balanced, nutrient-dense meals to support metabolic health and sustained energy.

Chapter 6

Lunch Recipes

Salads with a Twist

Quinoa Avocado Salad

Time: 10 minutes

Serves: 2

A refreshing mix of quinoa and avocado, packed with fiber and healthy fats.

Ingredients:

- 1 cup cooked quinoa
- 1 avocado, diced
- 1/2 cucumber, sliced
- 1/4 cup chopped parsley
- 1 tablespoon olive oil
- Juice of 1 lemon

Instructions:

1. Toss all ingredients in a bowl.
2. Drizzle with olive oil and lemon juice, and serve.

Citrus Kale Salad

Time: 10 minutes

Serves: 2

A vitamin-packed kale salad with citrus for a zesty twist.

Ingredients:

- 2 cups kale, chopped
- 1 orange, segmented
- 1/4 cup pomegranate seeds
- 1 tablespoon olive oil
- Juice of 1 lemon

Instructions:

1. Massage kale with lemon juice and olive oil.
2. Add orange segments and pomegranate seeds. Toss and serve.

Roasted Sweet Potato and Black Bean Salad

Time: 15 minutes

Serves: 2

Sweet potatoes and black beans make this salad hearty and satisfying.

Ingredients:

- 1 cup roasted sweet potatoes, diced
- 1/2 cup cooked black beans
- 1/2 red onion, sliced
- 1 tablespoon olive oil
- 1 teaspoon cumin

Instructions:

1. Toss roasted sweet potatoes and black beans with olive oil and cumin.
2. Serve over a bed of greens or as is.

Cucumber Mango Salad

Time: 10 minutes

Serves: 2

A refreshing salad combining cucumbers and mango with a tangy lime dressing.

Ingredients:

- 1 cucumber, diced
- 1 mango, diced
- 1/4 cup chopped cilantro
- Juice of 1 lime

Instructions:

1. Combine cucumber, mango, and cilantro in a bowl.
2. Drizzle with lime juice, toss, and serve.

Broccoli and Chickpea Salad

Time: 10 minutes

Serves: 2

A protein-packed salad with roasted broccoli and chickpeas.

Ingredients:

- 1 cup roasted broccoli
- 1/2 cup cooked chickpeas
- 1 tablespoon tahini (optional)
- 1 teaspoon lemon juice

Instructions:

1. Toss broccoli and chickpeas together.
2. Drizzle with lemon juice and optional tahini.

Spiralized Zucchini Salad

Time: 10 minutes

Serves: 2

A light, refreshing zucchini salad with a lemon vinaigrette.

Ingredients:

- 2 zucchinis, spiralized
- 1/2 cup cherry tomatoes, halved
- 1 tablespoon olive oil
- Juice of 1 lemon

Instructions:

1. Spiralize the zucchini and toss with tomatoes.
2. Drizzle with olive oil and lemon juice, and serve.

Watermelon and Cucumber Salad

Time: 10 minutes

Serves: 2

A cool, hydrating salad perfect for hot days.

Ingredients:

- 1 cup diced watermelon
- 1 cucumber, sliced
- 1/4 cup mint leaves, chopped
- Juice of 1 lime

Instructions:

1. Combine all ingredients in a bowl.
2. Toss gently and serve immediately.

Roasted Cauliflower Salad

Time: 15 minutes

Serves: 2

Roasted cauliflower paired with fresh greens and a light vinaigrette.

Ingredients:

- 1 cup roasted cauliflower
- 1/2 cup mixed greens
- 1 tablespoon olive oil
- 1 teaspoon apple cider vinegar

Instructions:

1. Combine roasted cauliflower and greens.
2. Drizzle with olive oil and apple cider vinegar. Toss and serve.

Beet and Carrot Salad

Time: 10 minutes

Serves: 2

A colorful, crunchy salad with fresh beets and carrots.

Ingredients:

- 1 beet, grated
- 1 carrot, grated
- 1/4 cup raisins
- 1 tablespoon olive oil

Instructions:

1. Toss grated beet and carrot with raisins.
2. Drizzle with olive oil and serve.

Avocado and Tomato Salad

Time: 10 minutes

Serves: 2

A simple, nutrient-dense salad with creamy avocado and fresh tomatoes.

Ingredients:

- 1 avocado, diced
- 1 cup cherry tomatoes, halved
- 1/4 cup chopped parsley
- Juice of 1 lemon

Instructions:

1. Toss avocado, tomatoes, and parsley in a bowl.
2. Drizzle with lemon juice and serve.

Hearty Grain Bowls

Quinoa and Veggie Bowl

Time: 10 minutes

Serves: 2

A filling bowl with quinoa, roasted veggies, and a lemon tahini dressing.

Ingredients:

- 1 cup cooked quinoa
- 1 cup roasted veggies (zucchini, bell peppers)
- 1 tablespoon tahini
- Juice of 1 lemon

Instructions:

1. Combine quinoa and roasted veggies in a bowl.
2. Drizzle with tahini and lemon juice. Toss and serve.

Brown Rice and Avocado Bowl

Time: 10 minutes

Serves: 2

Brown rice with creamy avocado and fresh veggies for a balanced bowl.

Ingredients:

- 1 cup cooked brown rice
- 1 avocado, diced
- 1/2 cucumber, sliced
- 1 tablespoon olive oil

Instructions:

1. Combine brown rice, avocado, and cucumber in a bowl.
2. Drizzle with olive oil and serve.

Millet and Roasted Veggie Bowl

Time: 10 minutes

Serves: 2

A fiber-rich millet bowl with roasted vegetables and a light dressing.

Ingredients:

- 1 cup cooked millet
- 1 cup roasted vegetables
- 1 tablespoon olive oil
- 1 teaspoon balsamic vinegar

Instructions:

1. Combine millet and roasted vegetables.
2. Drizzle with olive oil and balsamic vinegar. Serve warm or cold.

Wild Rice and Lentil Bowl

Time: 15 minutes

Serves: 2

A hearty bowl with wild rice and lentils for a high-protein meal.

Ingredients:

- 1 cup cooked wild rice
- 1/2 cup cooked lentils
- 1/4 cup chopped cilantro
- Juice of 1 lime

Instructions:

1. Combine wild rice, lentils, and cilantro in a bowl.
2. Drizzle with lime juice and serve.

Sorghum and Sweet Potato Bowl

Time: 15 minutes

Serves: 2

Sorghum paired with roasted sweet potatoes for a nutrient-dense, energizing bowl.

Ingredients:

- 1 cup cooked sorghum
- 1 cup roasted sweet potatoes
- 1 tablespoon olive oil
- 1 teaspoon smoked paprika

Instructions:

1. Combine sorghum and roasted sweet potatoes in a bowl.
2. Drizzle with olive oil and smoked paprika. Serve warm.

Buckwheat and Broccoli Bowl

Time: 15 minutes

Serves: 2

A gluten-free buckwheat bowl with roasted broccoli and a lemon vinaigrette.

Ingredients:

- 1 cup cooked buckwheat
- 1 cup roasted broccoli
- 1 tablespoon olive oil
- Juice of 1 lemon

Instructions:

1. Combine buckwheat and roasted broccoli.
2. Drizzle with olive oil and lemon juice. Serve warm.

Teff and Avocado Bowl

Time: 10 minutes

Serves: 2

A superfood bowl featuring teff, avocado, and fresh greens.

Ingredients:

- 1 cup cooked teff
- 1 avocado, sliced
- 1/2 cup spinach
- 1 tablespoon olive oil

Instructions:

1. Combine teff, avocado, and spinach.
2. Drizzle with olive oil and serve.

Amaranth and Carrot Bowl

Time: 15 minutes

Serves: 2

A protein-packed amaranth bowl with roasted carrots and a tangy dressing.

Ingredients:

- 1 cup cooked amaranth
- 1/2 cup roasted carrots
- 1 tablespoon tahini
- Juice of 1 lime

Instructions:

1. Combine amaranth and roasted carrots.
2. Drizzle with tahini and lime juice. Serve warm.

Farro and Spinach Bowl

Time: 10 minutes

Serves: 2

A hearty farro bowl with fresh spinach and a lemon dressing.

Ingredients:

- 1 cup cooked farro
- 1/2 cup spinach
- 1 tablespoon olive oil
- Juice of 1 lemon

Instructions:

1. Combine farro and spinach in a bowl.
2. Drizzle with olive oil and lemon juice. Serve warm.

Quinoa and Kale Bowl

Time: 10 minutes

Serves: 2

A nutrient-dense quinoa bowl with kale and roasted veggies.

Ingredients:

- 1 cup cooked quinoa
- 1/2 cup roasted kale
- 1 tablespoon olive oil
- Juice of 1 lime

Instructions:

1. Combine quinoa, kale, and roasted veggies.
2. Drizzle with olive oil and lime juice, and serve.

Quick Wraps and Sandwiches

Avocado and Veggie Wrap

Time: 5 minutes

Serves: 2

A simple and fresh avocado and veggie wrap that's both filling and nutritious.

Ingredients:

- 2 gluten-free wraps
- 1 avocado, mashed
- 1/2 cucumber, sliced
- 1/2 bell pepper, sliced
- 1/4 cup spinach leaves

Instructions:

1. Spread mashed avocado onto the gluten-free wraps.
2. Layer with cucumber, bell pepper, and spinach.

3. Roll up and serve immediately.

Roasted Veggie and Hummus Wrap

Time: 10 minutes

Serves: 2

A satisfying wrap filled with roasted vegetables and creamy hummus.

Ingredients:

- 2 gluten-free wraps
- 1/2 cup roasted vegetables (zucchini, bell peppers)
- 1/4 cup hummus
- 1/4 cup arugula

Instructions:

1. Spread hummus over the wraps.
2. Add roasted vegetables and arugula.
3. Roll up the wraps and serve.

Cucumber and Avocado Sandwich

Time: 5 minutes

Serves: 2

A light and refreshing sandwich with cucumber, avocado, and gluten-free bread.

Ingredients:

- 4 slices gluten-free bread
- 1 avocado, sliced
- 1/2 cucumber, sliced
- 1 tablespoon olive oil

Instructions:

1. Spread avocado slices on gluten-free bread.

2. Top with cucumber slices and drizzle with olive oil.

3. Serve open-faced or as a sandwich.

Turkey Lettuce Wrap

Time: 5 minutes

Serves: 2

A protein-packed lettuce wrap with turkey, avocado, and fresh veggies.

Ingredients:

- 4 large lettuce leaves
- 4 slices turkey breast (deli-style, nitrate-free)
- 1/2 avocado, sliced
- 1/4 cucumber, sliced

Instructions:

1. Lay the lettuce leaves flat and place a slice of turkey on each.

2. Add avocado and cucumber slices.

3. Roll up and serve immediately.

Chickpea Salad Wrap

Time: 10 minutes

Serves: 2

A flavorful chickpea salad wrap that's both filling and protein-rich.

Ingredients:

- 2 gluten-free wraps
- 1 cup cooked chickpeas, mashed
- 1 tablespoon tahini (optional)
- 1/4 cup shredded carrots

- 1/4 cup chopped parsley

Instructions:

1. Mash chickpeas with tahini (if using) until creamy.
2. Spread the chickpea mixture on the wraps.
3. Add carrots and parsley. Roll up and serve.

Tuna and Avocado Sandwich

Time: 5 minutes

Serves: 2

A gluten-free tuna salad sandwich made creamy with mashed avocado.

Ingredients:

- 4 slices gluten-free bread
- 1 can tuna in water, drained
- 1 avocado, mashed
- 1 tablespoon lemon juice

Instructions:

1. Mix the drained tuna with mashed avocado and lemon juice.
2. Spread the mixture on the gluten-free bread.
3. Serve as a sandwich or open-faced.

Falafel Lettuce Wraps

Time: 10 minutes

Serves: 2

These lettuce wraps feature homemade or store-bought falafel for a flavorful, plant-based meal.

Ingredients:

- 4 lettuce leaves
- 4 falafel patties

- 1/4 cup cucumber slices
- 1 tablespoon tahini (optional)

Instructions:

1. Place falafel patties inside the lettuce leaves.
2. Add cucumber slices and drizzle with tahini.
3. Wrap up and serve.

Roasted Sweet Potato and Spinach Wrap

Time: 10 minutes

Serves: 2

A warm and comforting wrap with roasted sweet potatoes and fresh spinach.

Ingredients:

- 2 gluten-free wraps
- 1 cup roasted sweet potato cubes
- 1/4 cup fresh spinach leaves
- 1 tablespoon olive oil

Instructions:

1. Fill each wrap with roasted sweet potatoes and spinach.
2. Drizzle with olive oil and roll up. Serve warm or cold.

Quinoa and Veggie Sandwich

Time: 10 minutes

Serves: 2

A high-protein, gluten-free sandwich featuring quinoa and fresh veggies.

Ingredients:

- 4 slices gluten-free bread

- 1/2 cup cooked quinoa
- 1/4 cup shredded carrots
- 1/4 cucumber, sliced

Instructions:

1. Spread quinoa on the gluten-free bread.
2. Add shredded carrots and cucumber slices.
3. Serve as an open-faced sandwich or regular sandwich.

Chicken and Avocado Wrap

Time: 10 minutes

Serves: 2

A satisfying chicken and avocado wrap, perfect for a quick meal.

Ingredients:

- 2 gluten-free wraps
- 1 cup cooked chicken breast, shredded
- 1/2 avocado, sliced
- 1/4 cup shredded lettuce

Instructions:

1. Lay out the wraps and layer with chicken, avocado, and lettuce.
2. Roll up the wraps and serve.

Chapter 7

Dinner Recipes

Grilled, Roasted, and Steamed Lean Proteins

Grilled Lemon Herb Chicken

Time: 20 minutes

Serves: 4

Juicy, marinated chicken breasts with lemon and fresh herbs, grilled to perfection.

Ingredients:

- 4 chicken breasts
- Juice of 2 lemons
- 2 tablespoons olive oil
- 1 tablespoon fresh rosemary, chopped

Instructions:

1. Marinate the chicken in lemon juice, olive oil, and rosemary for 30 minutes.
2. Grill over medium heat for 6-8 minutes per side until fully cooked. Serve hot.

Roasted Garlic Herb Salmon

Time: 25 minutes

Serves: 4

Oven-roasted salmon with garlic and herbs, perfect for a lean, high-protein dinner.

Ingredients:

- 4 salmon fillets
- 2 tablespoons olive oil
- 2 cloves garlic, minced

- 1 tablespoon fresh thyme

Instructions:

1. Preheat oven to 400°F (200°C).
2. Place salmon fillets on a baking sheet and drizzle with olive oil.
3. Sprinkle with garlic and thyme, and roast for 15-18 minutes until cooked through.

Steamed Cod with Lemon and Dill

Time: 15 minutes

Serves: 4

Delicate cod fillets steamed with fresh lemon and dill for a light, flavorful meal.

Ingredients:

- 4 cod fillets
- Juice of 1 lemon
- 1 tablespoon fresh dill, chopped

Instructions:

1. Place cod fillets in a steamer basket.
2. Drizzle with lemon juice and sprinkle with dill.
3. Steam for 10-12 minutes until fish flakes easily with a fork.

Grilled Turkey Breast

Time: 20 minutes

Serves: 4

Tender turkey breast grilled and seasoned with herbs for a lean protein option.

Ingredients:

- 4 turkey breast cutlets
- 2 tablespoons olive oil

- 1 tablespoon dried oregano

Instructions:

1. Brush turkey breasts with olive oil and season with oregano.
2. Grill over medium heat for 6-8 minutes per side. Serve immediately.

Roasted Chicken Thighs

Time: 30 minutes

Serves: 4

Succulent chicken thighs roasted with garlic and rosemary, perfect for a protein-rich dinner.

Ingredients:

- 4 bone-in chicken thighs
- 2 cloves garlic, minced
- 1 tablespoon fresh rosemary

Instructions:

1. Preheat oven to 400°F (200°C).
2. Place chicken thighs on a baking sheet, rub with garlic, and sprinkle with rosemary.
3. Roast for 25-30 minutes until crispy and golden.

Steamed Shrimp with Garlic and Lemon

Time: 10 minutes

Serves: 4

Quick and easy steamed shrimp with fresh garlic and lemon, perfect for a light dinner.

Ingredients:

- 1 lb shrimp, peeled and deveined
- 2 cloves garlic, minced
- Juice of 1 lemon

Instructions:

1. Steam shrimp for 5-7 minutes until pink and cooked through.
2. Toss with garlic and lemon juice, and serve immediately.

Grilled Pork Tenderloin

Time: 25 minutes

Serves: 4

Lean pork tenderloin marinated and grilled for a flavorful, protein-packed dinner.

Ingredients:

- 1 pork tenderloin
- 2 tablespoons olive oil
- 1 tablespoon Dijon mustard (optional)

Instructions:

1. Marinate the pork tenderloin in olive oil and mustard for 30 minutes.
2. Grill over medium heat for 10-12 minutes per side. Slice and serve.

Roasted Turkey Meatballs

Time: 25 minutes

Serves: 4

Turkey meatballs roasted in the oven for a simple, lean, protein-rich meal.

Ingredients:

- 1 lb ground turkey
- 2 cloves garlic, minced
- 1 tablespoon fresh parsley, chopped

Instructions:

- Preheat oven to 375°F (190°C).

- Mix ground turkey, garlic, and parsley in a bowl. Form into meatballs and place on a baking sheet.
- Roast for 20-25 minutes until cooked through.

Steamed Tilapia with Herbs

Time: 15 minutes

Serves: 4

A light and lean steamed tilapia dish, seasoned with fresh herbs.

Ingredients:

- 4 tilapia fillets
- 1 tablespoon fresh basil, chopped
- Juice of 1 lime

Instructions:

1. Steam tilapia for 10-12 minutes until fully cooked.
2. Drizzle with lime juice and sprinkle with basil before serving.

Grilled Lamb Chops

Time: 20 minutes

Serves: 4

Tender grilled lamb chops seasoned with garlic and rosemary.

Ingredients:

- 4 lamb chops
- 2 cloves garlic, minced
- 1 tablespoon fresh rosemary

Instructions:

1. Marinate lamb chops in garlic and rosemary for 30 minutes.

2. Grill over medium heat for 6-8 minutes per side. Serve hot.

Roasted Brussels Sprouts

Time: 20 minutes

Serves: 4

Crispy roasted Brussels sprouts, seasoned with olive oil and sea salt.

Ingredients:

- 2 cups Brussels sprouts, halved
- 2 tablespoons olive oil
- Salt and pepper to taste

Instructions:

1. Preheat oven to 400°F (200°C).
2. Toss Brussels sprouts with olive oil, salt, and pepper.
3. Roast for 18-20 minutes until crispy and golden.

Garlic Roasted Broccoli

Time: 20 minutes

Serves: 4

Roasted broccoli with garlic, a simple and nutrient-rich side dish.

Ingredients:

- 2 cups broccoli florets
- 2 cloves garlic, minced
- 1 tablespoon olive oil

Instructions:

1. Preheat oven to 400°F (200°C).
2. Toss broccoli with olive oil and garlic.
3. Roast for 15-20 minutes until tender.

Steamed Green Beans with Lemon

Time: 10 minutes

Serves: 4

Steamed green beans with fresh lemon juice for a light, refreshing side.

Ingredients:

- 2 cups green beans, trimmed
- Juice of 1 lemon

Instructions:

1. Steam green beans for 5-7 minutes until tender.
2. Drizzle with lemon juice and serve.

Roasted Sweet Potatoes

Time: 25 minutes

Serves: 4

Sweet potatoes roasted until caramelized, seasoned with olive oil and sea salt.

Ingredients:

- 2 large sweet potatoes, diced
- 2 tablespoons olive oil

Instructions:

1. Preheat oven to 400°F (200°C).
2. Toss sweet potatoes with olive oil and roast for 25-30 minutes until crispy.

Steamed Carrots with Ginger

Time: 10 minutes

Serves: 4

Lightly steamed carrots with a touch of fresh ginger.

Ingredients:

- 2 cups sliced carrots
- 1 tablespoon grated ginger

Instructions:

1. Steam carrots for 5-7 minutes until tender.
2. Toss with grated ginger and serve.

Roasted Cauliflower

Time: 20 minutes

Serves: 4

A crispy, flavorful roasted cauliflower dish, perfect as a side.

Ingredients:

- 1 head cauliflower, chopped
- 2 tablespoons olive oil

Instructions:

1. Preheat oven to 400°F (200°C).
2. Toss cauliflower with olive oil and roast for 20 minutes until golden.

Sautéed Spinach with Garlic

Time: 10 minutes

Serves: 4

A quick and easy spinach sauté with garlic, packed with nutrients.

Ingredients:

- 2 cups fresh spinach
- 2 cloves garlic, minced

Instructions:

1. Heat olive oil in a pan and sauté garlic for 1-2 minutes.
2. Add spinach and cook until wilted, about 3-4 minutes. Serve immediately.

Roasted Zucchini with Thyme

Time: 15 minutes

Serves: 4

Roasted zucchini with a hint of thyme, a light and flavorful side.

Ingredients:

- 2 zucchinis, sliced
- 1 tablespoon olive oil
- 1 teaspoon fresh thyme

Instructions:

1. Preheat oven to 400°F (200°C).
2. Toss zucchini with olive oil and thyme.
3. Roast for 15-18 minutes until tender.

Steamed Asparagus with Lemon

Time: 10 minutes

Serves: 4

Tender steamed asparagus with a squeeze of fresh lemon juice.

Ingredients:

- 1 bunch asparagus, trimmed
- Juice of 1 lemon

Instructions:

1. Steam asparagus for 5-7 minutes until tender.
2. Drizzle with lemon juice and serve.

Sautéed Mushrooms with Garlic

Time: 10 minutes

Serves: 4

A savory side of sautéed mushrooms with garlic, perfect for pairing with lean proteins.

Ingredients:

- 2 cups sliced mushrooms
- 2 cloves garlic, minced

Instructions:

1. Heat olive oil in a pan and sauté garlic for 1-2 minutes.
2. Add mushrooms and cook until browned, about 5-7 minutes. Serve hot.

Easy One-Pot Meals

One-Pot Chicken and Quinoa

Time: 30 minutes

Serves: 4

A hearty one-pot meal featuring chicken, quinoa, and fresh vegetables for a balanced, protein-packed dinner.

Ingredients:

- 4 chicken breasts, diced

- 1 cup quinoa, rinsed
- 2 cups vegetable broth
- 1 zucchini, diced
- 1 bell pepper, diced
- 2 cloves garlic, minced

Instructions:

1. Heat a tablespoon of olive oil in a large pot and sauté garlic until fragrant.
2. Add chicken and cook until browned.
3. Add quinoa, broth, and vegetables. Simmer for 20 minutes until quinoa is cooked and chicken is tender.

One-Pot Lentil and Vegetable Stew

Time: 35 minutes

Serves: 4

A nourishing stew made with lentils and a variety of vegetables, offering a filling and nutritious dinner.

Ingredients:

- 1 cup dried lentils, rinsed
- 1 carrot, diced
- 1 zucchini, diced
- 1 bell pepper, chopped
- 2 cloves garlic, minced
- 4 cups vegetable broth

Instructions:

1. In a large pot, sauté garlic in olive oil for 1-2 minutes.
2. Add lentils and vegetable broth. Bring to a boil, then reduce heat and simmer for 20 minutes.
3. Add vegetables and simmer for an additional 10 minutes until tender.

One-Pot Coconut Curry Chicken

Time: 30 minutes

Serves: 4

A rich coconut curry with tender chicken, sweet potatoes, and warming spices, all cooked in one pot.

Ingredients:

- 4 chicken thighs, diced
- 1 sweet potato, diced
- 1 can coconut milk
- 1 tablespoon curry powder
- 1/2 teaspoon turmeric

Instructions:

1. Heat oil in a pot and brown the chicken.
2. Add sweet potato, coconut milk, curry powder, and turmeric.
3. Simmer for 20 minutes until the chicken is fully cooked and the sweet potato is tender.

One-Pot Turkey and Cauliflower Rice Stir-Fry

Time: 25 minutes

Serves: 4

A healthy stir-fry with ground turkey and cauliflower rice, perfect for a quick and easy one-pot meal.

Ingredients:

- 1 lb ground turkey
- 4 cups cauliflower rice
- 1 zucchini, diced
- 1 bell pepper, diced

- 1 tablespoon olive oil

Instructions:

1. Heat olive oil in a large pan and cook ground turkey until browned.
2. Add cauliflower rice and vegetables, cooking until tender, about 10 minutes. Serve hot.

One-Pot Shrimp and Vegetable Paella

Time: 30 minutes

Serves: 4

A simple and flavorful gluten-free paella with shrimp, bell peppers, and peas.

Ingredients:

- 1 lb shrimp, peeled and deveined
- 1 cup short-grain rice
- 1 bell pepper, diced
- 1/2 cup peas
- 2 cups vegetable broth

Instructions:

1. Heat oil in a large pan and sauté bell peppers.
2. Add rice and broth, and simmer for 15 minutes.
3. Add shrimp and peas, cooking until the shrimp are pink and rice is tender.

One-Pot Beef and Sweet Potato Stew

Time: 40 minutes

Serves: 4

A warming stew with tender beef, sweet potatoes, and flavorful herbs, all cooked in one pot.

Ingredients:

- 1 lb beef stew meat, cubed

- 2 sweet potatoes, diced
- 1 onion, diced
- 2 cloves garlic, minced
- 4 cups beef broth

Instructions:

1. Brown beef in a large pot with olive oil.
2. Add garlic, onion, sweet potatoes, and broth.
3. Simmer for 30 minutes until the beef is tender and sweet potatoes are soft.

One-Pot Vegetable and Chickpea Stew

Time: 35 minutes

Serves: 4

A protein-packed chickpea stew loaded with vegetables for a filling, plant-based one-pot meal.

Ingredients:

- 1 can chickpeas, drained
- 1 zucchini, diced
- 1 carrot, sliced
- 2 cups spinach
- 4 cups vegetable broth

Instructions:

1. Sauté zucchini and carrots in olive oil in a large pot.
2. Add chickpeas, spinach, and broth. Simmer for 20 minutes until vegetables are tender. Serve hot.

One-Pot Salmon and Quinoa

Time: 30 minutes

Serves: 4

A healthy one-pot meal featuring salmon fillets and quinoa cooked with fresh vegetables.

Ingredients:

- 4 salmon fillets
- 1 cup quinoa, rinsed
- 2 cups vegetable broth
- 1 bell pepper, diced
- 1 zucchini, diced

Instructions:

1. Cook quinoa in vegetable broth in a large pot for 15 minutes.
2. Add salmon fillets and vegetables, cover, and simmer for another 10-12 minutes until the salmon is cooked through.

One-Pot Chicken and Vegetable Soup

Time: 30 minutes

Serves: 4

A light and comforting soup with chicken, vegetables, and fresh herbs.

Ingredients:

- 4 chicken breasts, shredded
- 1 carrot, diced
- 1 celery stalk, diced
- 4 cups chicken broth

Instructions:

1. Bring chicken broth to a boil and add vegetables.
2. Add shredded chicken and simmer for 20 minutes. Serve hot.

One-Pot Zucchini Noodles with Ground Beef

Time: 25 minutes

Serves: 4

A low-carb, high-protein one-pot meal featuring zucchini noodles and ground beef, perfect for an easy dinner.

Ingredients:

- 1 lb ground beef
- 4 zucchinis, spiralized
- 1 onion, diced
- 2 cloves garlic, minced

Instructions:

1. Brown the ground beef in a large pot with olive oil.
2. Add onions and garlic, cooking for 3-4 minutes.
3. Add zucchini noodles and cook for another 5 minutes until tender. Serve immediately.

Chapter 8

Snack Recipes

Quick, No-Bake Snacks

Coconut Date Energy Balls

Time: 10 minutes

Serves: 12 balls

Sweet and chewy, these coconut date energy balls are perfect for a quick energy boost.

Ingredients:

- 1 cup pitted dates
- 1/2 cup shredded coconut
- 1 tablespoon chia seeds

Instructions:

1. Blend dates and chia seeds in a food processor until smooth.
2. Roll into balls and coat with shredded coconut.
3. Chill for 30 minutes before serving.

Sunflower Seed Energy Balls

Time: 10 minutes

Serves: 12 balls

A nut-free energy ball made with sunflower seeds for a crunchy texture and protein boost.

Ingredients:

- 1 cup sunflower seeds
- 1/2 cup dried apricots
- 1 tablespoon flaxseed meal

Instructions:

1. Pulse sunflower seeds and apricots in a food processor.
2. Roll into balls and refrigerate for 30 minutes before enjoying.

Pumpkin Seed and Date Energy Balls

Time: 10 minutes

Serves: 12 balls

Energizing pumpkin seeds paired with sweet dates for a satisfying snack.

Ingredients:

*   1 cup pumpkin seeds
*   1 cup dates, pitted
*   1 tablespoon chia seeds

Instructions:

1. Blend all ingredients in a food processor until smooth.
2. Roll into balls and chill for 30 minutes before serving.

Coconut Lime Energy Balls

Time: 10 minutes

Serves: 12 balls

A zesty, tropical energy ball packed with lime and coconut.

Ingredients:

*   1 cup pitted dates
*   1/2 cup shredded coconut
*   Zest of 1 lime

Instructions:

1. Blend dates and lime zest in a food processor.

2. Roll into balls and coat with shredded coconut.

3. Chill before serving.

Chia and Apricot Energy Balls

Time: 10 minutes

Serves: 12 balls

A chewy and nutrient-dense energy ball combining chia seeds and dried apricots.

Ingredients:

- 1 cup dried apricots
- 1 tablespoon chia seeds
- 1/2 cup shredded coconut

Instructions:

1. Pulse apricots and chia seeds in a food processor.

2. Form into balls and coat with shredded coconut.

3. Refrigerate for 30 minutes before serving.

Cranberry Date Energy Balls

Time: 10 minutes

Serves: 12 balls

Tart cranberries and sweet dates make these energy balls deliciously balanced.

Ingredients:

- 1 cup pitted dates
- 1/2 cup dried cranberries
- 1 tablespoon flaxseed meal

Instructions:

1. Blend dates and cranberries in a food processor.

2. Roll into balls and chill for 30 minutes before serving.

Chocolate Coconut Energy Balls

Time: 10 minutes

Serves: 12 balls

A rich and satisfying snack made with raw cacao and coconut.

Ingredients:

- 1 cup pitted dates
- 1/2 cup shredded coconut
- 1 tablespoon raw cacao powder

Instructions:

1. Blend dates and cacao powder in a food processor.
2. Form into balls and coat with coconut.
3. Refrigerate before serving.

Carrot Cake Energy Balls

Time: 10 minutes

Serves: 12 balls

Sweet and spiced, these energy balls taste like a bite-sized version of carrot cake.

Ingredients:

- 1/2 cup shredded carrots
- 1 cup pitted dates
- 1/2 teaspoon cinnamon

Instructions:

1. Blend shredded carrots, dates, and cinnamon in a food processor.
2. Roll into balls and chill before serving.

Cinnamon Raisin Energy Balls

Time: 10 minutes

Serves: 12 balls

These cinnamon-spiced energy balls are made with raisins for natural sweetness.

Ingredients:

- 1 cup raisins
- 1/2 teaspoon cinnamon
- 1/4 cup shredded coconut

Instructions:

1. Pulse raisins and cinnamon in a food processor.
2. Form into balls and roll in shredded coconut.
3. Chill for 30 minutes before serving.

Orange Date Energy Balls

Time: 10 minutes

Serves: 12 balls

Bright and citrusy, these energy balls are perfect for a refreshing snack.

Ingredients:

- 1 cup pitted dates
- Zest of 1 orange
- 1 tablespoon flaxseed meal

Instructions:

1. Blend dates and orange zest in a food processor.
2. Roll into balls and refrigerate before serving.

Baked Zucchini Chips

Time: 25 minutes

Serves: 4

Crispy baked zucchini chips, a healthy and light alternative to traditional chips.

Ingredients:

- 2 zucchinis, thinly sliced
- 1 tablespoon olive oil

Instructions:

1. Preheat oven to 400°F (200°C).
2. Toss zucchini slices with olive oil.
3. Arrange on a baking sheet and bake for 20-25 minutes until crispy.

Sweet Potato Chips

Time: 30 minutes

Serves: 4

Thin, crispy sweet potato chips that are baked, not fried, for a healthy snack.

Ingredients:

- 2 sweet potatoes, thinly sliced
- 1 tablespoon olive oil

Instructions:

1. Preheat oven to 375°F (190°C).
2. Toss sweet potato slices with olive oil.
3. Spread on a baking sheet and bake for 25-30 minutes until crispy.

Kale Chips

Time: 15 minutes

Serves: 4

Crispy, nutrient-dense kale chips with a light crunch, perfect for snacking.

Ingredients:

- 1 bunch kale, torn into bite-sized pieces
- 1 tablespoon olive oil

Instructions:

1. Preheat oven to 350°F (175°C).
2. Toss kale with olive oil.
3. Spread on a baking sheet and bake for 10-15 minutes until crispy.

Carrot Chips

Time: 20 minutes

Serves: 4

Baked carrot chips with a hint of sweetness and crunch.

Ingredients:

- 3 large carrots, thinly sliced
- 1 tablespoon olive oil

Instructions:

1. Preheat oven to 375°F (190°C).
2. Toss carrot slices with olive oil.
3. Bake for 15-20 minutes until crispy.

Beet Chips

Time: 25 minutes

Serves: 4

Naturally sweet and earthy, these beet chips are baked to crispy perfection.

Ingredients:

- 2 large beets, thinly sliced
- 1 tablespoon olive oil

Instructions:

1. Preheat oven to 375°F (190°C).
2. Toss beet slices with olive oil.
3. Arrange on a baking sheet and bake for 20-25 minutes until crispy.

Butternut Squash Chips

Time: 25 minutes

Serves: 4

Lightly crispy butternut squash chips for a flavorful, healthy snack.

Ingredients:

- 1 butternut squash, thinly sliced
- 1 tablespoon olive oil

Instructions:

1. Preheat oven to 375°F (190°C).
2. Toss squash slices with olive oil.
3. Bake for 20-25 minutes until crispy.

Parsnip Chips

Time: 25 minutes

Serves: 4

Crunchy baked parsnip chips, a perfect gluten-free alternative to regular chips.

Ingredients:

- 2 parsnips, thinly sliced
- 1 tablespoon olive oil

Instructions:

- Preheat oven to 375°F (190°C).
- Toss parsnip slices with olive oil.
- Spread on a baking sheet and bake for 20-25 minutes until crispy.

Eggplant Chips

Time: 25 minutes

Serves: 4

Crispy, savory eggplant chips that are light and full of flavor.

Ingredients:

- 1 large eggplant, thinly sliced
- 1 tablespoon olive oil

Instructions:

1. Preheat oven to 400°F (200°C).
2. Toss eggplant slices with olive oil.
3. Bake for 20-25 minutes until crispy.

Turnip Chips

Time: 25 minutes

Serves: 4

A healthy twist on chips using turnips for a crunchy, fiber-rich snack.

Ingredients:

- 2 turnips, thinly sliced
- 1 tablespoon olive oil

1. Preheat oven to 375°F (190°C).
2. Toss turnip slices with olive oil.
3. Spread on a baking sheet and bake for 20-25 minutes until crispy.

Cucumber Chips

Time: 15 minutes

Serves: 4

Thin, crunchy cucumber chips for a refreshing and healthy snack.

Ingredients:

- 2 cucumbers, thinly sliced
- 1 tablespoon olive oil

Instructions:

1. Preheat oven to 375°F (190°C).
2. Toss cucumber slices with olive oil.
3. Bake for 10-15 minutes until crispy.

Homemade Trail Mix

Pumpkin Seed Trail Mix

Time: 5 minutes

Serves: 4

A crunchy mix of pumpkin seeds, dried cranberries, and coconut flakes.

Ingredients:

- 1/2 cup pumpkin seeds
- 1/4 cup dried cranberries

- 1/4 cup coconut flakes

Instructions:

1. Mix all ingredients in a bowl and serve.

Sunflower Seed and Raisin Trail Mix

Time: 5 minutes

Serves: 4

A simple trail mix combining sunflower seeds and raisins for a quick, energy-packed snack.

Ingredients:

- 1/2 cup sunflower seeds
- 1/4 cup raisins

Instructions:

2. Mix all ingredients and store in an airtight container.

Coconut and Date Trail Mix

Time: 5 minutes

Serves: 4

A naturally sweet trail mix with chewy dates, coconut flakes, and seeds.

Ingredients:

- 1/2 cup chopped dates
- 1/4 cup shredded coconut
- 1/4 cup pumpkin seeds

Instructions:

3. Mix all ingredients in a bowl.
4. Store in an airtight container and enjoy as a quick snack.

Cranberry and Sunflower Seed Trail Mix

Time: 5 minutes

Serves: 4

A tart and sweet trail mix packed with cranberries, sunflower seeds, and coconut flakes.

Ingredients:

- 1/2 cup dried cranberries
- 1/4 cup sunflower seeds
- 1/4 cup coconut flakes

Instructions:

1. Combine all ingredients in a bowl.
2. Store in an airtight container for snacking on the go.

Date and Apricot Trail Mix

Time: 5 minutes

Serves: 4

A chewy, fruity trail mix that combines chopped dates, dried apricots, and pumpkin seeds.

Ingredients:

- 1/4 cup chopped dates
- 1/4 cup dried apricots, chopped
- 1/4 cup pumpkin seeds

Instructions:

1. Mix dates, apricots, and seeds in a bowl.
2. Store in an airtight container and enjoy anytime.

Coconut and Raisin Trail Mix

Time: 5 minutes

Serves: 4

A simple, crunchy trail mix with shredded coconut and raisins for a quick energy boost.

Ingredients:

- 1/4 cup shredded coconut
- 1/2 cup raisins
- 1/4 cup pumpkin seeds

Instructions:

1. Combine all ingredients and mix well.
2. Store in an airtight container for easy snacking.

Pumpkin Seed and Dried Apple Trail Mix

Time: 5 minutes

Serves: 4

A refreshing trail mix featuring dried apples and crunchy pumpkin seeds.

Ingredients:

- 1/4 cup dried apple slices, chopped
- 1/2 cup pumpkin seeds
- 1/4 cup shredded coconut

Instructions:

1. Mix the dried apple slices, pumpkin seeds, and coconut together in a bowl.
2. Store in an airtight container.

Sunflower Seed and Dried Blueberry Trail Mix

Time: 5 minutes

Serves: 4

A unique trail mix combining the sweetness of dried blueberries with crunchy sunflower seeds.

Ingredients:

- 1/4 cup dried blueberries
- 1/2 cup sunflower seeds
- 1/4 cup coconut flakes

Instructions:

1. Combine all ingredients in a bowl.
2. Mix well and store in an airtight container for snacking.

Apricot and Raisin Trail Mix

Time: 5 minutes

Serves: 4

A chewy and fruity mix with dried apricots and raisins, great for quick snacks.

Ingredients:

- 1/4 cup chopped dried apricots
- 1/2 cup raisins
- 1/4 cup sunflower seeds

Instructions:

1. Mix all ingredients in a bowl.
2. Store in an airtight container.

Pumpkin Seed and Date-Coconut Trail Mix

Time: 5 minutes

Serves: 4

A tasty blend of pumpkin seeds chopped dates, and coconut flakes for a crunchy yet chewy trail mix.

Ingredients:

- 1/4 cup chopped dates
- 1/4 cup pumpkin seeds
- 1/4 cup coconut flakes

Instructions:

- Combine all ingredients in a bowl.
- Store in an airtight container and enjoy as a portable snack.

Chapter 9

Dessert Recipes

Low-Sugar Sweets

Coconut Bliss Bites

Time: 10 minutes

Serves: 12 bites

A light, coconut-flavored treat that's naturally sweetened and guilt-free.

Ingredients:

- 1 cup shredded coconut
- 1/4 cup coconut oil, melted
- 1 tablespoon maple syrup (optional)

Instructions:

1. Mix shredded coconut, coconut oil, and maple syrup in a bowl.
2. Form into small balls and refrigerate for 30 minutes before serving.

Chia Seed Pudding

Time: 10 minutes (plus chilling)

Serves: 2

A creamy, nutritious pudding sweetened with a touch of fruit and perfect for a light dessert.

Ingredients:

- 3 tablespoons chia seeds
- 1 cup coconut milk
- 1/2 teaspoon vanilla extract
- 1 tablespoon maple syrup (optional)

Instructions:

1. Mix chia seeds, coconut milk, vanilla extract, and maple syrup in a jar.
2. Stir well and refrigerate for at least 2 hours, stirring occasionally. Serve chilled.

Banana Oat Cookies

Time: 15 minutes

Serves: 12 cookies

Simple, healthy cookies made with ripe bananas and oats for a naturally sweet treat.

Ingredients:

- 2 ripe bananas, mashed
- 1 cup rolled oats
- 1/2 teaspoon cinnamon

Instructions:

1. Preheat oven to 350°F (175°C).
2. Mix mashed bananas, oats, and cinnamon.
3. Drop spoonfuls onto a baking sheet and bake for 12-15 minutes.

Coconut Chocolate Bites

Time: 10 minutes

Serves: 12 bites

A low-sugar, rich chocolate treat with the goodness of coconut.

Ingredients:

- 1/2 cup shredded coconut
- 2 tablespoons raw cacao powder
- 2 tablespoons coconut oil, melted

Instructions:

1. Mix shredded coconut, cacao powder, and coconut oil.
2. Form into small balls and chill for 30 minutes before serving.

Date Energy Bars

Time: 10 minutes

Serves: 8 bars

Naturally sweet date bars with seeds, perfect for a light dessert or snack.

Ingredients:

- 1 cup pitted dates
- 1/4 cup sunflower seeds
- 1 tablespoon chia seeds

Instructions:

1. Blend all ingredients in a food processor until smooth.
2. Press the mixture into a baking dish, refrigerate for 1 hour, then cut into bars.

Coconut Macaroons

Time: 15 minutes

Serves: 12

Light, airy macaroons made with shredded coconut and just a touch of sweetness.

Ingredients:

- 1 cup shredded coconut
- 2 tablespoons maple syrup
- 1 teaspoon vanilla extract

Instructions:

1. Preheat oven to 350°F (175°C).
2. Mix all ingredients together and form into small balls.

3. Place on a baking sheet and bake for 10-12 minutes.

Baked Cinnamon Apples

Time: 20 minutes

Serves: 4

Sweet baked apples with cinnamon, a simple and naturally sweet dessert.

Ingredients:

- 4 apples, cored and sliced
- 1 teaspoon cinnamon
- 1 tablespoon maple syrup (optional)

Instructions:

1. Preheat oven to 350°F (175°C).
2. Place apple slices in a baking dish, sprinkle with cinnamon, and drizzle with maple syrup.
3. Bake for 20 minutes.

Coconut and Berry Parfait

Time: 10 minutes

Serves: 2

Layers of coconut cream and fresh berries for a naturally sweet, low-sugar dessert.

Ingredients:

- 1/2 cup coconut cream
- 1/2 cup mixed berries
- 1 teaspoon vanilla extract

Instructions:

1. Layer coconut cream and berries in a glass.
2. Top with a drizzle of vanilla extract and serve chilled.

Pumpkin Spice Bites

Time: 10 minutes

Serves: 12 bites

Guilt-free pumpkin spice bites with a hint of cinnamon and natural sweetness.

Ingredients:

- 1/2 cup pumpkin puree
- 1 cup shredded coconut
- 1/2 teaspoon cinnamon

Instructions:

1. Mix pumpkin puree, shredded coconut, and cinnamon.
2. Form into small balls and refrigerate for 30 minutes before serving.

Coconut Vanilla Ice Cream

Time: 5 minutes (plus freezing)

Serves: 4

A simple, dairy-free ice cream made with coconut milk and vanilla for a low-sugar dessert.

Ingredients:

- 1 can full-fat coconut milk
- 1 teaspoon vanilla extract
- 2 tablespoons maple syrup (optional)

Instructions:

1. Blend coconut milk, vanilla extract, and maple syrup.
2. Pour into a freezer-safe container and freeze for 2-3 hours, stirring every hour.

Grilled Pineapple with Lime

Time: 10 minutes

Serves: 4

Juicy grilled pineapple with a splash of lime, offering natural sweetness.

Ingredients:

- 1 pineapple, sliced
- Juice of 1 lime

Instructions:

1. Grill pineapple slices for 2-3 minutes on each side.
2. Drizzle with lime juice and serve warm.

Baked Pears with Cinnamon

Time: 20 minutes

Serves: 4

Sweet baked pears topped with cinnamon for a light and healthy dessert.

Ingredients:

- 4 pears, halved
- 1 teaspoon cinnamon

Instructions:

1. Preheat oven to 350°F (175°C).
2. Place pear halves in a baking dish, sprinkle with cinnamon, and bake for 20 minutes.

Mango Sorbet

Time: 5 minutes (plus freezing)

Serves: 4

A refreshing, naturally sweet mango sorbet that's perfect for hot days.

Ingredients:

- 2 ripe mangoes, peeled and chopped
- 1/4 cup coconut water

Instructions:

1. Blend mangoes and coconut water in a food processor until smooth.
2. Freeze for 2-3 hours and serve.

Apple Slices with Coconut Cream

Time: 5 minutes

Serves: 4

Simple apple slices served with a dollop of coconut cream for a light dessert.

Ingredients:

- 4 apples, sliced
- 1/2 cup coconut cream

Instructions:

1. Arrange apple slices on a plate and top with coconut cream.
2. Serve immediately.

Strawberry Banana Popsicles

Time: 5 minutes (plus freezing)

Serves: 6

Naturally sweetened popsicles made with strawberries and bananas.

Ingredients:

- 1 banana, sliced
- 1 cup strawberries, hulled

Instructions:

1. Blend strawberries and bananas in a food processor until smooth.
2. Pour into popsicle molds and freeze for 3 hours.

Baked Plums with Coconut

Time: 15 minutes

Serves: 4

Soft baked plums topped with shredded coconut for a naturally sweet dessert.

Ingredients:

- 4 plums, halved
- 1/4 cup shredded coconut

Instructions:

1. Preheat oven to 350°F (175°C).
2. Place plums in a baking dish and sprinkle with shredded coconut.
3. Bake for 12-15 minutes.

Berry Salad with Lime

Time: 5 minutes

Serves: 4

A refreshing berry salad with a hint of lime for added brightness.

Ingredients:

- 1 cup strawberries, sliced
- 1 cup blueberries
- Juice of 1 lime

Instructions:

1. Toss the berries with lime juice in a bowl.
2. Serve chilled for a refreshing treat.

Grilled Pineapple

Ingredients:

- 1 pineapple, sliced into rounds
- 1 tablespoon coconut sugar
- 1 teaspoon cinnamon

Instructions:

1. Sprinkle pineapple slices with coconut sugar and cinnamon.
2. Grill each side for 2-3 minutes until caramelized.
3. Serve warm with a drizzle of lime juice.

Raspberry Coconut Cream Cups

Ingredients:

- 1 cup raspberries
- 1 cup coconut cream
- 1 tablespoon maple syrup
- 1 teaspoon vanilla extract

Instructions:

1. Whip coconut cream with maple syrup and vanilla extract.
2. Layer raspberries and coconut cream in small cups.
3. Chill for 30 minutes before serving.

Citrus Salad with Mint

Ingredients:

- 2 oranges, segmented

- 1 grapefruit, segmented
- 1 tablespoon fresh mint, chopped
- 1 teaspoon maple syrup

Instructions:

1. Combine orange and grapefruit segments in a bowl.
2. Add chopped mint and drizzle with maple syrup.
3. Toss lightly and chill before serving.

Conclusion

Living the Good Energy Lifestyle is a commitment to long-term health and well-being, and maintaining the momentum is as crucial as beginning the journey. Achieving balance requires consistent effort in both physical and mental health, as this lifestyle isn't about perfection but building a sustainable routine. The tips provided in the Good Energy Recipe Book offer practical ways to stay on track and motivated for the long haul.

Maintaining balance means understanding that habits take time to become second nature, but once you commit, the benefits are transformative. As discussed in the book, following key habits like consistent movement, mindful eating, and stress management will lead to sustained energy levels and overall well-being. Keeping track of your habits, reflecting on barriers, and using an accountability partner can help keep you engaged with your goals. Whether it's logging your food, scheduling nature time, or incorporating movement into social activities, these strategies help create a healthy routine that sticks .

A powerful insight from the Good Energy Recipe Book is that staying consistent doesn't mean being rigid. Life will throw curveballs, but being adaptable in your approach helps maintain balance. If you fall off the wagon, reset by picking a habit that excites you and start small. Whether you're working on your fitness goals, improving sleep, or refining your diet, focusing on progress over perfection is essential .

Staying motivated for the long term often comes down to understanding your "why." Knowing why you want to live a healthier life, beyond just looking or feeling good, helps anchor your efforts. The Good Energy Recipe Book emphasizes the importance of aligning your lifestyle choices with your deeper values, like having the energy to be present for loved ones or respecting the environment by choosing sustainable food options.

Building a sustainable routine means creating habits that fit seamlessly into your life. Habit stacking—like adding a few minutes of movement after a daily routine—can make new habits easier to maintain. Using habit-forming techniques, such as setting triggers and attaching rewards, turns small actions into significant lifestyle changes over time . Celebrate the small wins and remember that every healthy choice brings you closer to living a vibrant, energized life.

Incorporating accountability systems, like having a partner to check in with or scheduling activities that align with your Good Energy habits, ensures that motivation remains high. Prepaying for wellness classes, organizing healthy social activities, and making wellness part of your daily environment are all ways to reinforce your commitment to your health journey .

Living the Good Energy Lifestyle is not just about following a set of rules—it's about creating a life that feels energizing, fulfilling, and aligned with your values. By building a routine that supports your health goals and staying motivated through habit-forming strategies, you can enjoy sustained energy and well-being. The journey may not be linear, but with the tools and insights from the Good Energy Recipe Book, you have everything you need to create lasting change and live your healthiest life.